Morning
Rituals

Also by Leslie Koren
Love Rituals
Restorative Rituals

Morning
Rituals

IDEAS AND INSPIRATION
TO GET ENERGIZED

LESLIE KOREN

ARTISAN | NEW YORK

This book is intended as a reference volume only, not as a medical manual. The information
given here is for educational and informational purposes only. All forms of exercise carry
some level of inherent risk—if you have any concerns about the exercises in this book,
please consult a physician before attempting any of the poses or sequences. The authors and
publisher are not responsible for any loss, damage, or injury to any person or entity caused
directly or indirectly by the information contained in this book.

Library of Congress Cataloging-in-Publication Data

Names: Koren, Leslie, author.
Title: Morning rituals : ideas and inspiration to get energized / Leslie Koren.
Description: New York, NY : Artisan, a division of Workman Publishing Co.,Inc., [2021]
Identifiers: LCCN 2021014926 | ISBN 9781648290299 (hardcover)
Subjects: LCSH: Mind and body. | Inspiration. | Exercise.
Classification: LCC BF151 .K67 2021 | DDC 158.1—dc23
LC record available at https://lccn.loc.gov/2021014926

Design by Heitman-Ford + Co.

Artisan books are available at special discounts when purchased in bulk for premiums and
sales promotions as well as for fund-raising or educational use. Special editions or book
excerpts also can be created to specification. For details, contact the Special Sales Director at
the address below, or send an e-mail to specialmarkets@workman.com.

For speaking engagements, contact speakersbureau@workman.com.

Published by Artisan
A division of Workman Publishing Co., Inc.
225 Varick Street
New York, NY 10014-4381
artisanbooks.com
Artisan is a registered trademark of Workman Publishing Co., Inc.

Published simultaneously in Canada by Thomas Allen & Son, Limited

Printed in China
First printing, October 2021

10 9 8 7 6 5 4 3 2 1

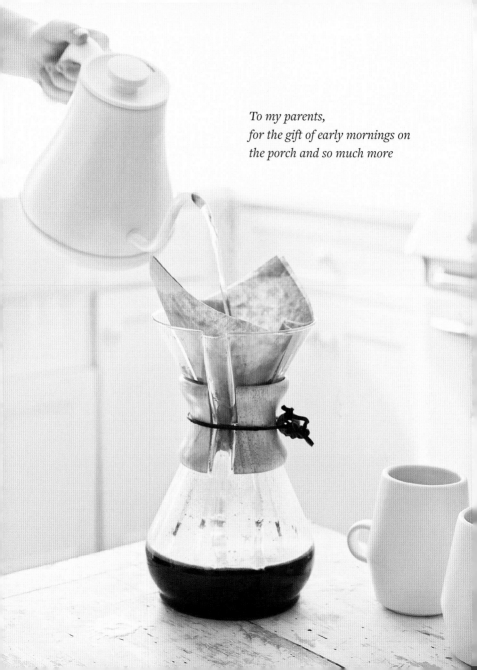

To my parents,
for the gift of early mornings on
the porch and so much more

Contents

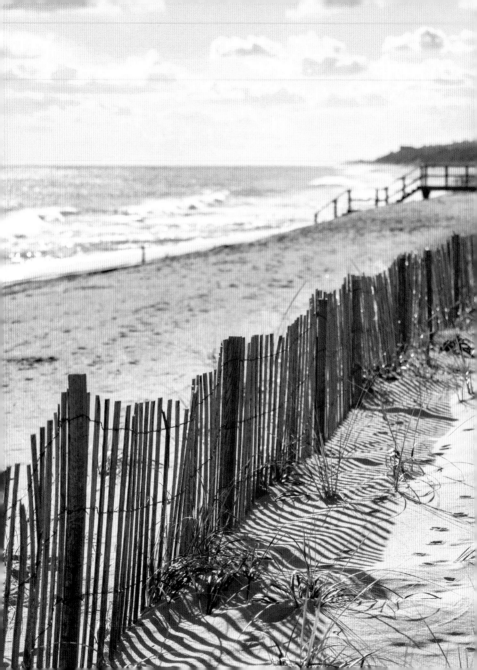

Introduction

During a particularly challenging time, my family started taking the same walk on the same city beach every Sunday morning. We didn't set out to create a new routine—we just knew we needed to exchange our house for a new setting, to get out into nature. And yet, after about a month of these regular walks, we started calling them our "beach ritual."

Some mornings we struggled to make it happen: a kid who didn't want to get in the car, jackets that weren't warm enough, a mom who moved too slowly (at least according to everyone else in my family!). But because it was now an official family ritual, we always set off and, one way or another, we were always rewarded. Sometimes there were tangible goodies, like the treasure trove of sea glass we collected one morning after a storm. But more often the gifts were soulful— the feeling of connection that follows a good walk-and-talk, or the sense of expansiveness that comes from watching waves roll in and out. Ours wasn't the most beautiful beach in the world, but it was good enough when we started and beyond special after our umpteenth return. A not-insignificant bonus: The rest of our Sunday, and really our week, got immeasurably better, too.

That's the power of ritual, and that's what this book is all about. It's designed to help you build rituals into your mornings, each and every day, because the very act of deciding to do something on repeat in an intentional and meaningful way will enrich your day and your life. It's a claiming and reclaiming of what matters to you. It sounds simple, but it has profound reverberations.

Many people think rituals need to involve grand gestures or they won't "count," but that raises the question of who, exactly, decides what counts? To me, a ritual has value if it makes my existence better. Period. Even small acts, I've found, can make a big difference.

And that's what you'll find on the following pages: powerful—but doable!—rituals that will elevate the first hours of your day and help you feel centered, energized, and ready to take on the world. Of course, I don't anticipate you'll do every ritual in this book every morning—that would be a lot. I recognize that time is a luxury, especially on workdays. Fortunately, you don't need to wake at dawn or have hours on hand to incorporate worthwhile rituals into your morning. Several of the suggestions that follow are meant to enhance the things you already do every day. I've purposefully included rituals that you can perform while tending to responsibilities, like starting work—only now you'll do them with an added boost! Others will bring new elements to your routine. Certainly, embrace those ideas that immediately grab your attention. But I encourage you to also try some that don't initially appeal, because you might be surprised by what they provide.

Here's another secret to incorporating rituals into your morning: You don't have to commit to any of these ideas forever. Some may work for you during a specific time and place in your life, while others will be longer lasting. So consider this permission (if you need it) to weave in the rituals that are beneficial to you in a given moment, and let them go when they stop serving you. I've often included different suggestions for how you might go about each one, as a way to encourage you to customize these rituals to your own wants and needs. Much like creative cooks can go into the kitchen and whip up a satisfying meal without relying on a recipe, I want you to feel empowered to improvise and create rituals that benefit you.

From the moment I wake up, and in almost every part of my life, I rely on rituals to help me be a happier and more grounded human, not to mention a more fulfilled partner, parent, daughter, colleague, and friend. And that's what I wish for you tomorrow morning, as the sun rises, the birds chatter, and so much possibility lies ahead. Whether your house is filled with calm or chaos, I hope you'll find rituals that nourish a more meaningful and energizing connection with your body and spirit, one that will carry you through the remaining hours of the day.

Getting Started and Keeping Going

There are many ideas on the following pages, but there is no one right way to incorporate rituals into your morning. The goal is to find a path that's sustainable and enjoyable *for you*. If you're unsure where to begin, here are a few places to dive in.

Identify the sticky parts of your morning. Do you wish you ate a more nutritious breakfast? Or could get in some exercise? Or that you actually enjoyed your commute? There's a ritual for that (on pages 16, 61, and 98 respectively).

Pick a theme. Perhaps you want to focus on creativity, in which case I suggest writing morning pages (page 54), taking a walk (page 58), or reading a poem (page 70)— all different ways to get the juices flowing. If you wish to be energized, then unplug earlier (page 27), do calisthenics upon waking (page 46), take an invigorating shower (page 74), or listen to an anthem (page 91). Other possible themes: mindfulness, movement, nourishment. It's yours to choose.

Find a ritual buddy. As written, most of the rituals in this book are designed for you to do on your own. But you can and should incorporate other people in your life as desired. Performing these rituals with your kids, a partner, and/or friends is enriching in a different, also wonderful way. And it could keep you (and your companion) accountable: talk through your experiences, share wins, and note your challenges.

Let fate decide. Close your eyes and quickly flip through the pages—then stop at random. Commit to doing whichever ritual you landed on for the next week. If you like that experience, surprise yourself again and again, through both which ritual you'll do and the gifts it will bring to your life.

Identify existing rituals. You may find that you already have a meaningful ritual (or two) embedded in your morning routine, but you just haven't acknowledged it as such. If that is indeed the case, lean into the ritual, really owning that you've done this for yourself, and then consider what other complementary rituals you might like to incorporate into your day.

Start Your Morning the Night Before

There's a choose-your-own-adventure spirit to many of the rituals in this book, but the one thing I urge you to do is consider how much sleep you need to feel good in the morning and do everything in your power to give yourself that rest. If you wake up exhausted, your morning won't be what you had hoped, no matter how many rituals you incorporate. Plus, the more often you press snooze, the more likely you'll be to skip rituals in the rush to get out the door on time. The ideas on the following pages are designed to set you up for a good night's sleep and an energetic morning.

Prepping Tomorrow's Breakfast

One reason I love to incorporate small(ish) rituals into my days—and encourage you to do the same—is that they make life easier and lead to smart choices that also feel good. Case in point: preparing breakfast the night before. It's a small(ish) act of self-care that has a big impact. Waking up every morning to something nutritious (and delicious!) means you'll be less likely to grab a coffee shop pastry or skip breakfast altogether. You start the day on better footing, with more energy and at least one nourishing decision already under your belt.

As much as I delight in waking up to a premade breakfast, I also enjoy the late-night prepping. That's why the ritual is sustainable—it's not just a gift to my future self, but it's also gratifying in the moment. Unlike the urgency that creeps up while cooking dinner, the process of prepping overnight oats or chia pudding or 7½-minute eggs is calming and meditative. I wait until everyone else is in bed so I'm alone in the kitchen, cue up a podcast episode I've been saving, and start tinkering. I purposely keep the stakes low, preparing the same few breakfasts again and again (often in batches to set myself up for the week) so there's no stress about mishaps. I've even come to enjoy the tidying afterward, a quick wipe of the counter that satisfies the part of me that's ready to wrap up the day (and makes my morning return extra pleasant).

Overnight Oats

This supereasy alternative to hot oatmeal takes just a few minutes to whip up and is an energizing way to kick off the day. Whole-grain oats help control blood sugar and reduce bad cholesterol. Plus they are delicious—especially in this creamy, chewy, slightly sweet breakfast. Grab it from the fridge in the morning and mix in whatever extras you'd like. SERVES 1

½ cup (45 g) old-fashioned rolled oats

½ to 1 cup (120 to 240 ml) milk or milk alternative (such as oat or coconut milk), depending on your preferred consistency

Small pinch of kosher or sea salt

OPTIONAL ADD-INS, FOR SERVING:

Spoonful of nut butter

Chopped nuts

Berries (fresh, or thawed if frozen) or grated apple

Dried fruit

Coconut flakes

Sweetener, like honey or maple syrup

Mix the oats, milk, and salt in a jar or resealable container. Store in the fridge overnight. In the morning, uncover and stir. Top with any desired add-ins and enjoy.

7½-Minute Eggs

Boiling eggs for 7½ minutes results in the perfect mix of jammy yolks and cooked whites. You can eat them plain, with just a sprinkle of salt and pepper; for a heartier, dressed-up version, I like to chop them, add avocado and a dash of Dijon mustard, and eat with crackers. SERVES 1

2 eggs (cold from the fridge)
Flaky sea salt and freshly cracked black pepper, for serving
Crackers (optional, for serving)

Fill a pot with enough water to cover the eggs and heat to a rolling boil. Gently lower the eggs into the water using a slotted spoon and cook for 7½ minutes. Meanwhile, prepare a bowl of ice water.

Using the slotted spoon, quickly transfer the eggs into the ice bath to stop the cooking. Take them out after they've cooled slightly, about 5 minutes. You can leave them on the counter overnight, if you prefer to eat them at room temperature, or put them in the refrigerator if you plan to eat them later in the week.

In the morning, peel the eggs, halve, and eat them with a sprinkling of salt and pepper, plain or with crackers.

Apple-Berry Chia Pudding

Chia seeds, which originate in Latin America, are rich in fiber, protein, calcium, and omega-3 fatty acids. You can sprinkle them on yogurt or other foods or make them into a pudding by soaking them in liquid (milk, milk alternatives, and juice are most common) for an hour or longer. This apple-berry version is a filling morning meal, and just calling it a pudding makes it seem like you're eating dessert for breakfast! **SERVES 1**

¼ cup (50 g) chia seeds

1 cup (240 ml) milk or milk alternative
   (such as oat or coconut milk)

½ cup (75 g) berries (fresh, or thawed if frozen)

¼ teaspoon (1 ml) vanilla extract

¼ cup (45 g) diced apple, or more, for serving

Sweetener, like honey or maple syrup, for serving (optional)

Whisk the chia seeds, milk, berries, and vanilla in a bowl until combined. Store in a jar or resealable container in the fridge overnight. In the morning, give the mixture a quick stir and add the apple and sweetener, if desired, to taste.

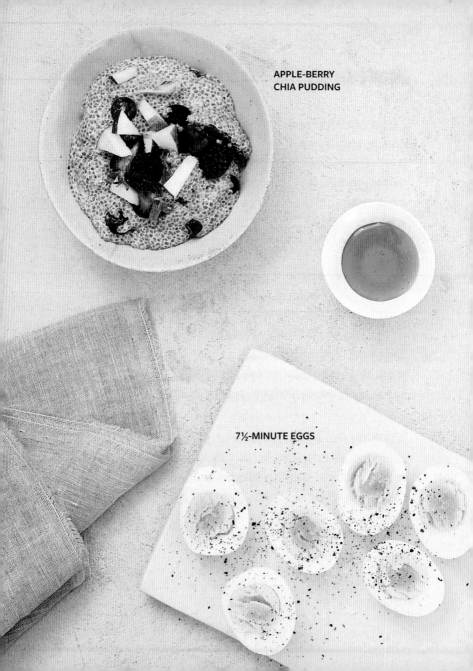

APPLE-BERRY
CHIA PUDDING

7½-MINUTE EGGS

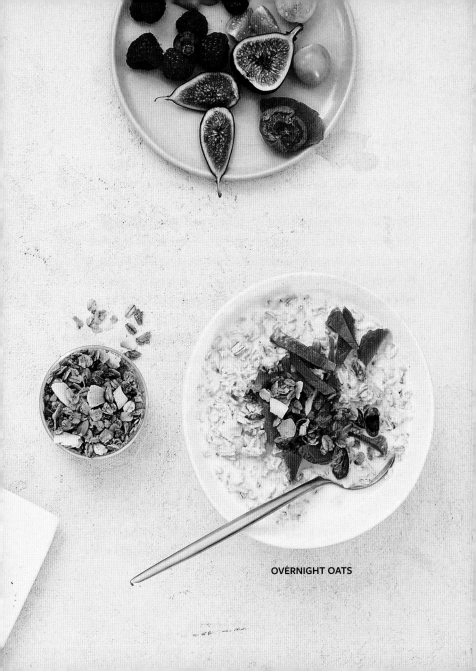

OVERNIGHT OATS

Relaxing with Essential Oils

People have turned to aromatherapy, and the essential oils at the heart of the treatment, for thousands of years. These oils, or highly concentrated plant liquids, are made by extracting the "essence" from flowers, leaves, stalks, fruits, and the like. Ancient Egyptians put them in cosmetics; traditional Chinese and Indian healers turned them into medicine. Today, essential oils are used for everything from relieving headaches to cleaning floors to boosting moods to—drumroll, please— getting a good night's rest. The latter use is particularly noteworthy because scent is the only one of the five senses that remains "active" while we sleep, and it travels directly to the parts of our brain tied to emotion and memory.

I'd like to say it's much easier to experiment with essential oils now than in, say, 3000 BCE, but I've also stood before rows and rows of essential oils on display, put off by the very modern problem of decision paralysis. Too many choices often make it harder to choose at all. For an easier time drifting off and sweeter dreams once you do, here are a few good places to start:

Bergamot. This delicate plant from southern Italy is thought to be a hybrid of lemon and bitter oranges. The slightly spicy citrus and floral aroma is both uplifting and calming, and it's a favorite of the perfume industry. Use it to de-stress and relax.

Chamomile. There are two popular versions of this herbal essential oil: Roman and German. You want the former, which has been used for ages for its soothing qualities. The calming scent is a sweet, fruity, and herbaceous mix.

Lavender. This purple flower's popular scent is a bedtime classic. The sweet floral aroma is an antidote to insomnia and anxiety.

Valerian. Another ancient medicinal herb well known for its ability to calm nerves, valerian has an earthy, woodsy aroma that's admittedly not for everyone. But if you like it, it's an excellent balm for any late-night worries or troubles falling asleep.

An essential oil ritual works on two levels: It sends a signal to your body and mind that it's time to let go of the day, and it encourages a (scientifically proven) sounder sleep. I regularly put a few drops of one of the above oils into a diffuser, along with some water, before bedtime. (This is great for kids' rooms, too; but do be careful with pets, as some essential oils are toxic to cats and dogs.) For similar results, you can also try the roll-on oil or pillow mist recipes that follow.

Bergamot Roll-On Oil

Never apply an essential oil directly to your skin because it might cause a bad reaction. Instead, make this simple, fragrant massage oil to dab on your pressure points before going to sleep. **MAKES ENOUGH TO FILL ONE ¼-OUNCE (7 ML) ROLLER BOTTLE**

10 drops bergamot essential oil

One ¼-ounce (7 ml) roller bottle or other small container

½ teaspoon (2 ml) vitamin E oil

1 teaspoon (5 ml) carrier oil, such as grapeseed, jojoba, sunflower, or apricot kernel

Put the bergamot oil into the bottle.

Add the vitamin E oil (it will prolong the life of your massage oil and feels nice on the skin). Fill the bottle with your carrier oil. Shake to combine. Test to see if the scent is strong enough; if you want more, add 1 or 2 drops of bergamot at a time, shake, and test until you're happy with the result.

Lavender Essential Oil Pillow Mist

Spray this mist on your pillow and sheets before getting into bed.

Spray bottle

Lavender essential oil

Vodka or unscented witch hazel

Distilled water

Fill your bottle about one-third full of vodka. Add 10 drops of lavender essential oil per ounce (30 ml) of liquid in your bottle; add up to 5 more drops, until the scent is to your desired strength. Top off the bottle with distilled water. Place the cap back on and shake for 20 seconds to combine. Give it another quick shake before spraying.

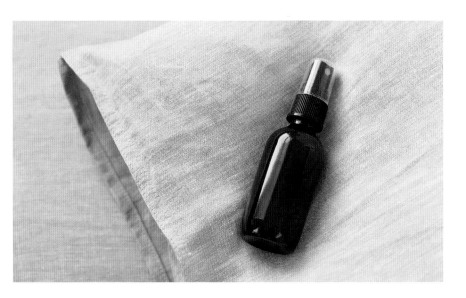

Planning Ahead

Because my day is significantly better if I exercise early in the morning, I make a ritual of piling my workout clothes by my bedside every night before sleep. That way, when I push back the covers the next morning, all I have to do is change and head downstairs. This is what habit-making experts call "removing friction points." I find it's helpful when I'm trying to achieve goals, like staying fit, and when I just want things to go more smoothly in general.

To eliminate obstacles from your morning, think about what you want or need to accomplish the next day and set yourself up for success before getting into bed. Maybe you want to prepare for your morning rituals—putting your journal and pen on the table for morning pages (see page 54) or organizing the food in your fridge so you can pack your lunch (see page 94). Or maybe you'll just make a ritual of reviewing the day ahead and planning accordingly. If you have an early meeting, for example, you might pick out your clothes, making sure everything is wrinkle-free and looks good together. It'll feel much better than trying on and discarding a million shirts as you race to get out of the house on time.

Whatever you choose to prep, think of it as an opportunity to care for yourself—a way to set the tone for both a restful night's sleep and a breezier morning.

Unplugging

I heard the loud boom of the falling tree during the last gasp of the daylong summer storm at my family's house in the country. Suddenly we lost power and any connection to the internet or phone lines. All devices rendered useless, I simply put them aside for the evening and luxuriated in the uninterrupted and unscrollable time by thumbing through magazines, taking a twilight walk, and eating a relaxed, candlelit dinner. If only it were always so easy to unplug!

I know, just as you probably do, that looking at screens before bed messes with my body's internal clock (its natural circadian rhythms), making it harder to fall asleep and stay asleep. But I still find it difficult to resist technology's allure. After all, these devices are designed to stimulate the brain's pleasure sensor. And they start us on a vicious cycle, because they also emit blue light that suppresses the production of melatonin, the hormone that makes us tired, so we're tempted to stay up even later, getting too few hours of the all-important REM sleep and waking up groggy and less energized.

But just as rituals can be employed to smooth out the early-morning hours, they can also ease the path to them. This ritual is simple but offers clear guidelines, so that once it becomes routine, the decisions that follow are effortless: Each night, one hour before bed, put your devices into their charging stations, then turn to something lo-fi and relaxing.

I always begin this transition to my quieter, device-free hour with a cup of mint tea. Truthfully, the reward felt a little lame at first—traveling down internet rabbit holes produced a lot more dopamine than an herbal brew—but I kept at it, and before long teatime became the cherished moment when I could pivot from doing to almost done. Sometimes you have to force a ritual for a while.

Think of this as your sacred nightly ritual: an hour to do what you want, with no pressure to respond to texts or emails. Perhaps you relish getting lost in a book or want to write in a journal at bedtime. Maybe you'll take a long, luxurious bath. You can carve out this hour for a hobby—drawing or knitting or solving a newspaper crossword puzzle. I love cooking, so I'll often get into bed with a cookbook and browse for inspiration. The point is, this is special "me time" that you've just reclaimed from the tech giants, and it's yours to spend as you wish.

A Calming Bedtime Breath

If you still struggle to fall asleep after your hour of screen-free downtime, try this 4-7-8 breathing exercise from Andrew Weil, MD, a bestselling author and pioneer of integrative medicine. I find it much more effective than counting backward from one hundred or worrying about how tired I'll be in the morning if I don't nod off quickly. The practice gains strength with day-over-day repetition; its effects might feel subtle on the first few tries but will become more pronounced the more nights you have under your belt.

1. Inhale through your nose for a mental count of four.

2. Hold your breath for a count of seven.

3. Exhale through your mouth for a count of eight.

4. Repeat one to three times.

Wake Up

Rise and shine! It's a new day and you're here for it, opening your eyes to the bright promise ahead. Unfurl those covers and meet the moment. As my beloved grandfather taught me: The early bird gets the worm. Let these rituals fill you with vim and vigor—goodness and possibility await.

Drinking Lemon Water

Perhaps, like me, you've heard somewhere in your wellness wanderings that a prebreakfast glass of lemon water is the answer to many of your "problems": that it will reset your digestive system, detoxify your body, trim your fat, make your skin glow. Not surprisingly, as with so many health fads, it turns out that experts don't find a squeeze of citrus *quite* that effective. Yet here I am recommending that you drink a glass of lemon water every morning anyway—but for a different reason entirely.

Think of this ritual as a little promise to yourself. Because the very acts of remembering to buy lemons, then waking up, rolling the lemon on the counter (which makes it extra juicy), cutting it in half, squeezing it into your glass or mug, pouring in the water (at your desired temperature), and staring out the window as you drink it could very well set you on the right path for whatever lies ahead.

As you go about this brief routine, I encourage you to forgo your phone or the news and, instead, consider how you want to care for yourself throughout the day. Perhaps, like my friend Claudia, you'll make it a moment for appreciation; while filling her kettle and turning on the stove, she gives thanks for the clean water and flowing gas—luxuries she doesn't take for granted after living through devastating fire seasons in California.

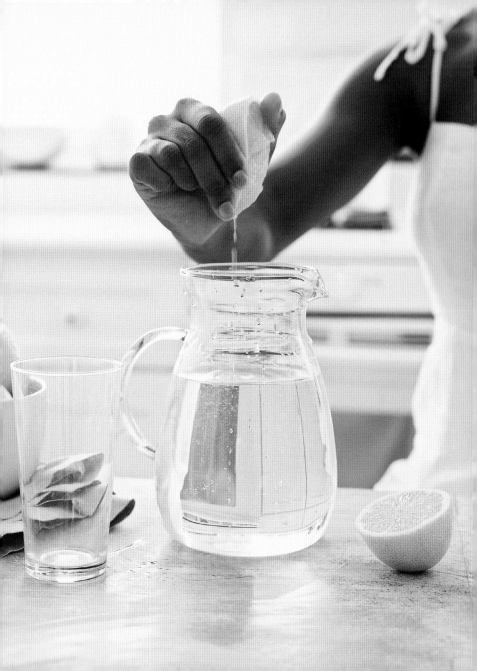

Breathing Deeply

Take a deep breath. Inhale through your nose, noticing how your belly and chest rise. Exhale through your mouth, watching your torso lower. Repeat this a few times, deeply imbibing that wondrous oxygen. Close your eyes if you want, or put your hand on your belly or chest to really feel the movement of your breath. You will take more than seventeen thousand breaths today, and the vast majority will go unnoticed. Let these first ones fully nourish you.

For something we do so automatically and regularly, breathing can be surprisingly challenging. As soon as we get scared, we hold our breath; when we're anxious, our breath becomes shallow, the air moving in and out from the shoulders rather than the diaphragm. But if we regularly start to pay attention to even just a few breaths a day, we gain a life-changing tool. Our breath connects us to ourselves: our emotions and our inner landscape. With minimal effort and a little know-how, it can relax, invigorate, and heal us. This age-old insight is found across many cultures and traditions, from the Chinese to the Greeks to early yoga practitioners.

For your morning breathing ritual, I recommend a few rounds of Lion's Breath, a pranayama exercise (meaning it comes from the yogic tradition) that is somehow both calming and awakening. The breathing technique relieves tension in your face and jaw and releases negative energy throughout your body. It's also great for building confidence.

1 Sit in a cross-legged position or on a chair. Rest your hands on your thighs.

2 Take a few even breaths to settle yourself and prepare.

3 Inhale deeply through your nose.

4 As you slowly exhale, open your mouth as wide as possible and stick out your tongue, curling the tip down toward your chin. Open your eyes wide as well and look up to the sky. Make a *haaaah* sound as the breath leaves your body.

5 Repeat two or three times.

Setting an Intention

There's a practice, rooted in Buddhism, of setting a morning intention. It's a quick but powerful way to touch base with your aspirations—not what you hope to accomplish before lunch but rather how you aim to experience the coming day's actions and encounters. Thupten Jinpa, PhD, founder of the Compassion Institute and a trained monk, explains it nicely in his book *A Fearless Heart*: "Like music, intention can influence our mood, thoughts, and feelings—setting an intention in the morning, we set the tone for the day."

So how can you begin this ritual tomorrow morning? First, set yourself up for success with a reminder wherever you first look after waking. Then ask yourself: *What is my intention for the day?* If your mind goes blank, that's fine. Time and practice make it easier, as does remembering that this isn't about nailing it. (In the beginning I worried that I would set the "wrong" intention and all would be lost—the mind can really play games.)

A few deep breaths will help you get quiet, so you can listen for any answers that bubble up. For me, some days the response is quite clear, telling me to connect to my body or to be less judgmental. Jinpa writes that he sometimes doesn't hear any answer. Same here, but I never regret asking the question.

Saluting the Sun

People have been waking up at dawn to do yoga for hundreds of years. One classic form is Surya Namaskar, or Sun Salutation, which is a series of eleven poses. The whole series is performed several times in a row, building heat in your body so that the tight, resistant parts on round 1 become looser by round 5 and maybe a little elastic by round 10-plus. Our physical and emotional experiences are linked, so your mood expands as well, nourished by the deep breaths and synchronized movements. Like all those other practitioners across time and place, you'll find yourself becoming stronger, calmer, more grounded, and just generally better at coping with whatever comes your way.

Of course, for all the legions who've made this a morning ritual, there are countless yogis who can't find their way onto their mats every morning, much as they may want to. But you can—if you don't already—by simply laying out your yoga mat, standing tall in Tadasana (Mountain Pose), and doing just one round of the series. For instructions, turn the page—but know that this is just one version of Surya Namaskar, and you should modify the poses as needed to feel good for you and your body (one source I suggest is *Every Body Yoga*; see page 102).

Surya Namaskar (Sun Salutation)

1 Start by standing tall in Tadasana (Mountain Pose), the crown of your head reaching for the sky, palms together in front of your heart.

2 Inhale as you raise your hands and gaze to the sky to greet the sun for Urdhva Hastasana (Upward Salute).

3 Exhale and bend forward at the hips, placing your hands on the floor in Uttanasana (Standing Forward Bend). If your hands don't reach the floor, bend your knees until you can touch the ground.

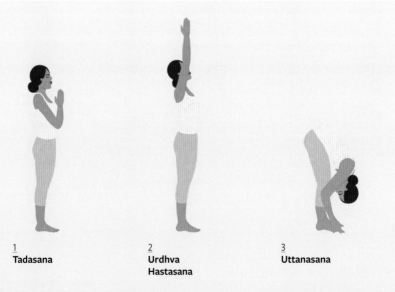

1
Tadasana

2
Urdhva Hastasana

3
Uttanasana

4   Inhale and extend your chin, chest, and crown of your head
     forward, while gazing at the floor. Keep your fingertips on
     the floor or on your shins with your legs strong. This is Ardha
     Uttanasana (Half Standing Forward Bend).

5   Exhale and step back to a plank (the top of a pushup), then
     bend your elbows and lower your body halfway to the ground for
     Chaturanga Dandasana (Four-Limbed Staff Pose).

6   Roll over your toes until the tops of your feet are pressing on
     the ground, then inhale and move your torso forward as you
     straighten your arms into Urdhva Mukha Svanasana (Upward-
     Facing Dog). When you get into the position, draw your shoulders
     back to open your chest.

continued

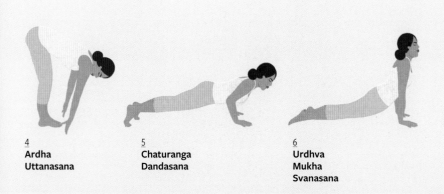

4
**Ardha
Uttanasana**

5
**Chaturanga
Dandasana**

6
**Urdhva
Mukha
Svanasana**

7   Exhale, tuck your toes under, and push your hips back and up, keeping your arms straight for Adho Mukha Svanasana (Downward-Facing Dog). Spread your fingers and press your knuckle joints down into the floor.

8   Inhale and step or jump your feet forward, lengthen your spine forward, and extend your chin, chest, and crown of your head forward again, while gazing at the floor, for Ardha Uttanasana (Half Standing Forward Bend).

9   Exhale back into Uttanasana (Standing Forward Bend) by bending at the hips and softening your spine.

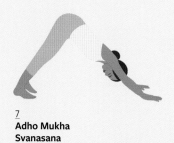

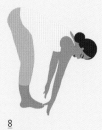

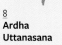

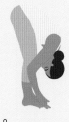

7
**Adho Mukha
Svanasana**

8
**Ardha
Uttanasana**

9
Uttanasana

10 Inhale and rise up, reaching for the sun and sky with both arms into another Urdhva Hastasana (Upward Salute).

11 Exhale as you lower your hands, placing them together at your heart for the return to Tadasana (Mountain Pose). Press your feet strongly into the floor to root yourself, feel the energy pulsing through your body, and raise your hands to begin another round, if you so desire.

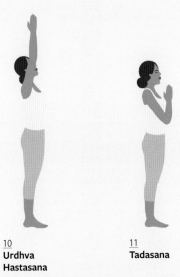

10
**Urdhva
Hastasana**

11
Tadasana

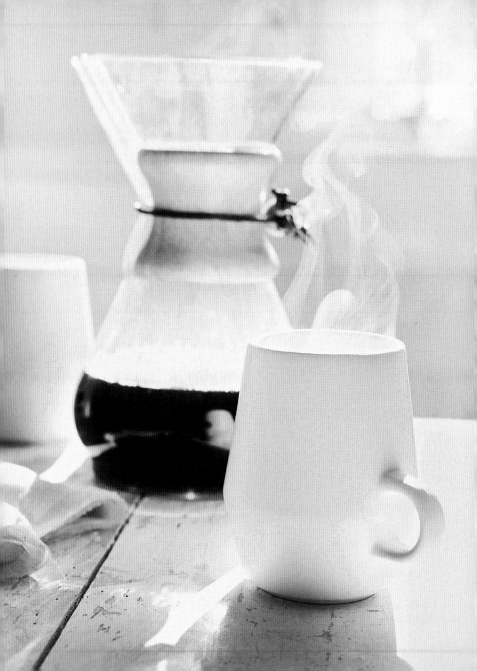

Savoring Your Coffee (or Tea)

When we first met, my now-husband and I operated at very different speeds: I was a whirling dervish, he preferred a slower pace. So he was aghast at my morning coffee "ritual," which consisted of picking up a watery cup of joe and an energy bar at the bodega and consuming both while driving through bumper-to-bumper traffic en route to my job as a crime reporter. And I had absolutely no patience for his, in which he boiled water to pour into a French press and let the grounds steep for several minutes before savoring his mug at the kitchen table.

His ritual added tremendous pleasure to his life, whereas my routine was merely a caffeine-delivery mechanism. Thankfully, I've since come around to his way of thinking. The more I tasted the moments of joy that arose from being deliberate, the more of them I wanted. They made my daily life feel richer, in a way I used to think could come only from big things like promotions or vacations.

At some point my coffee ritual became a tea ritual, which became a loose-leaf tea ritual—a small extra effort resulting in a better drink. And sourcing my tea is now a ritual of its own. Every time I pass through San Francisco's airport after visiting my brother, for example, I add time for a stop at the Samovar Tea House for a cherished bag of their English Breakfast. It's also led me to a kooky little tea-spice-and-British-crisps shop in my neighborhood, where I love the variety of teas as much as the eccentric owner loves Day of the Dead skeletons. It's the exponential math of rituals: added layers, added deliciousness.

Now every morning I place my tea infuser into the pink-striped mug my younger daughter painted for me—it's a treasure that ups the special factor. Likewise, I use a thin-neck kettle my oldest friend bought for me because she knew I cherish teatime. You don't need sentimental (or expensive) gear to make your daily cuppa, but having equipment you love does make it more luxurious.

While I still can't bear to wait the four recommended minutes for optimal brewing (some things never change), I sit at the counter and drink my tea slowly(ish), enjoying the soothing taste of the first sip, the warmth of the mug in my always-cold hands, and the quiet stillness before I kick into high gear. I recommend you, too, find a favorite spot to drink: in a cozy nook by a window, perhaps, or outside if the weather or space allows.

Caffeine Hits That Lend Themselves to Ritual

Your beverage of choice matters less than the thought you put into the making and drinking it, but these slow, lo-fi processes are well suited to conscious consumption.

- Letting coffee grounds steep for four minutes before plunging down the top of a French press

- Measuring loose-leaf tea into a strainer and steeping

- Vigorously whisking matcha, a ground green tea, into a froth

- "Blooming," or quickly prewetting, the coffee grounds and watching them expand before pouring in the remainder of the water for a pour-over coffee

- Carefully listening for the moment the brew starts gurgling while using an Italian moka pot

Doing Calisthenics

I once interviewed the legendary *Cosmopolitan* editor Helen Gurley Brown in her Manhattan office, in anticipation of the reissue of her groundbreaking book *Sex and the Single Girl*. Gurley Brown famously shocked early-1960s society by telling women to have lots of "nookie"—and to enjoy it! Amid leopard print wall-to-wall carpet, pink walls, and a needlepoint pillow with her motto "Good girls go to heaven, bad girls go everywhere," she told me about turning down marriage proposals, paying for a Mercedes-Benz with five thousand dollars in cash, and her devotion to morning rituals, chief among them the calisthenics set she completed every single day, even at eighty-one. Apparently leg lifts were a favorite move.

Over the many intervening years, I thought often of Gurley Brown's calisthenics ritual. Perhaps because, as she sat before me in lace stockings, an almost mini-dress, and pointy-toed slingbacks, she attributed her continued vitality to doing the exercises. Or perhaps because Gurley Brown, though her feminist legacy is a bit complicated, impressed my young self as a woman who had lived life on her own terms, beginning the moment she stepped out of bed.

A lot of people categorize exercise as a chore. If you are one of those folks, see if focusing on, and appreciating, your strength and ability to move shifts that mind-set. Recognizing what your body is able to accomplish might stop your brain from rebelling against something it has to do and give it a more positive association. Also, gratitude will help minimize the focus on achieving a "goal" and keep you grounded in the experience and your body.

The routine that follows is courtesy of Kirkland Shephard, a brilliant personal trainer in New York City. Shephard recommends that you perform the two warm-up movements to get the blood flowing, and then do each exercise for forty-five seconds—working up to ninety as you get stronger. But even doing just one exercise, such as holding a plank for thirty seconds every morning, is a perfectly wonderful ritual. Please modify as needed, or swap in other exercises that work for you; the spirit of this isn't to hold your plank endlessly but rather to move your body in whatever way builds strength, feels good, and ups your heart rate.

Warm-Ups

1 **Trunk twists:** Stand tall with your feet slightly wider than hip-width apart. Gently twist from side to side with your arms in a lazy (or passive) position. As the torso and hips open up, increase the range of the twist.

2 **Arm circles:** Stand tall with your feet slightly wider than hip-width apart and extend your arms so they are parallel with the floor. Begin with small circles in one direction and gently increase to larger circles as the shoulders warm up. After 20 or 30 seconds do the same thing in the opposite direction.

Calisthenics

1 **Plank:** Start in a tabletop position with your hands under your shoulders. Extend one leg back along the floor at a time. With your arms and legs straight, engage your core muscles and gaze slightly forward. Try not to hyperextend your elbows, so that your shoulder and arm muscles can fully engage.

2 **Push-ups:** Start in a plank and lower your body to the ground by bending your elbows—this can be done with your hands on a table if you are building strength. You can also modify by dropping your knees to the floor or starting with just half-reps, in which your chest doesn't go all the way down to the floor. Two form tips: First, try not to shrug your shoulders when you go down, and second, you're in proper alignment if your thumbs are just outside of your midchest line when you reach the floor.

3 **Squats:** Stand with your feet slightly wider than your shoulders, toes pointing out. Engage your core and squat down, bending your knees to slightly higher than 90 degrees, with the weight in your heels. Push off with your toes to return to your starting position, extending your legs, arms, and torso all the way up to maximize the movement.

4 **Jumping jacks:** Stand up with your legs together and your arms down at your sides. Bend your knees and jump into the air, stretching your arms overhead and spreading your legs out to shoulder width. Jump back to the starting position and repeat.

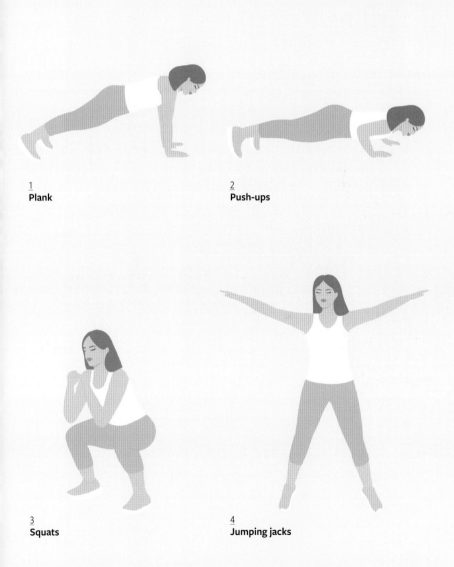

1
Plank

2
Push-ups

3
Squats

4
Jumping jacks

Feeling Grateful

The emerging science of happiness is a wonderful reminder of human progress. Twenty-five years ago, the field didn't exist; today it's a booming discipline, with Nobel Prize–winning researchers exploring what makes individuals and communities thrive. It turns out that while, yes, many of us must contend with tricky brain chemistry and challenging circumstances, there's lots we can do to feel more fulfilled, joyous, and satisfied. Cultivating gratitude is chief among those actions. By actively appreciating our good fortune, we counteract our brain's tendency to compare and despair. Shifting the focus to what we have, rather than what we lack, overrides our negativity bias. And while it's nice to notice broad gifts like health and home, happiness scientists have found that the practice works best when you're more specific. So, for example, today I'm grateful for the busy chirping of the baby birds that just hatched in the birdhouse under the Japanese maple tree, as well as for their watchful parents who get nervous when I pass too close by.

There's no right way to do this, so you can adopt any of the suggestions that follow or use a mix of these methods throughout your week.

Keep a gratitude journal. When you wake up, write down three things you're grateful for from the day before. For a twenty-first-century spin, consider texting a gratitude list to yourself (or using your notes app) so you have a running tally on your phone, or creating a private Instagram account to capture daily moments of gratitude.

Write a thank-you note or text. Be sincere in your gratitude, and, most important, send it! Researchers found too many people fret over the perfect wording and thus opt out. Don't fall into that trap, because the study discovered that following through made the recipient much happier than the letter writer anticipated (and the sender also got a big boost).

Share your gratitude list with someone. Take a few moments each morning to tell a partner, friend, or family member what you're appreciating. For example, each person in my household shares three moments of gratitude at dinner every night. It's a ritual that helps us share in one another's happiness.

Land in
Yourself

Soon you'll go off to your day and all it entails: work and play, good fortune and hardship, excitement and frustration. Before the busyness sets in, take a moment to reconnect with yourself and your surroundings and build a strong, stabilizing foundation so that you're ready for whatever awaits. These rituals will propel you all day long, giving you the gift of greater clarity, creativity, and purpose.

Writing Morning Pages

You know how everyone says to do "X" because it will make your life so much better, but no matter how hard you try you never manage to make it happen? Well, my X was writing a journal, a decades-long failed effort that dates back to a mostly blank grade-school Ziggy notebook I recently found in my parents' attic. At some point in adulthood, I decided I just wasn't a journal person and I gave up. Forever.

Or so I thought, until the day I read that author Elizabeth Gilbert writes three longhand pages when she wakes up, inspired by the morning-pages exercise in Julia Cameron's *The Artist's Way*. The idea made my heart skip, but then I thought, *Too bad I'm not a journal person*. A week later, I looked up from my seat on the train and saw a man across from me reading *The Artist's Way*. I'm pretty stubborn, but it felt like the universe was insisting. So the next morning I woke at dawn and sat down on the sofa to write three longhand pages. And I've done the exact same thing nearly every day since, at home or on vacation, on days I couldn't wait to put pen to paper and those when I dreaded it. I often write about the negative nonsense that clutters my thoughts. Sometimes I'll write lines of a poem I love. Other entries are filled with details of interactions or outings or thoughts or feelings. It doesn't really matter. What matters is that I have made a ritual of it, which changed a pathway in my brain and wrote over all the negative roadblocks I had about journaling. Which is pretty amazing, since journaling has made me happier and calmer and saner than I ever could have imagined—and I hope it will do the same for you. Here's how to get started:

1 When choosing your journal, avoid the "make it nice" trap. We're always pressured to make things look pretty for others, and I hope this space will be the opposite of that—a place for lovely thoughts, yes, but also for those that are messy and challenging. If you feel a special journal would make you *less* inclined to express a full range of emotions, then pick anything else—a spiral notebook, a pad, the plainest journal you can find.

2 As soon as possible after waking up, sit somewhere private and start writing, not stopping until you've completed a set number of longhand pages. Per Julia Cameron's advice I do three, but the number is up to you.

3 Write anything, without censoring yourself. As Cameron says, there is no wrong way to write morning pages. If you're stumped, try writing "I don't know what to write" or "blah blah blah" and chances

are you'll quickly find yourself writing something more substantive.

4 Stop yourself at your set number of pages, even if you're tempted to keep going. This limit is an essential part of the ritual and may be the thing that will keep you coming back day after day.

An important addendum: I strongly believe that a journal is a private space for one's own thoughts, and I encourage you to do whatever you can to create that privacy. I keep my current journal in the bottom of a bag no one in my house looks through, and I store the old ones high up in my closet (I've considered getting a lockbox!). I've even asked my husband to dispose of them if something happens to me.

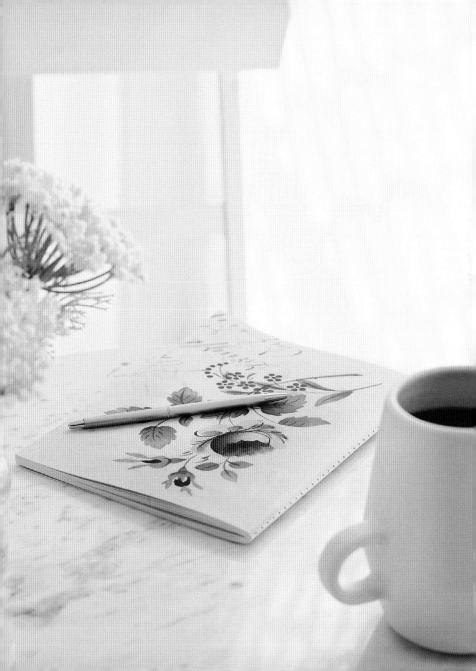

Taking a Walk . . .

Walking is a top five joy for me. When I'm older and freer of daily responsibilities, I hope to traverse the world's great pilgrimage paths, from the Camino de Santiago in Europe to Kumano Kodo in Japan. For now, though, I make do with walking in Brooklyn, which isn't a bad fate. On lucky mornings that means a twenty-minute walk to my older daughter's middle school. She's old enough to travel alone, but she lets me accompany her on Tuesdays and Thursdays, a generous move in these teen years that I don't take for granted. The rest of my day is infinitely better for having stepped out so early—there's a feeling of clarity and balance that's missing on the days I don't have a morning walk. This isn't about exercising, even though walking is great for our bodies. This ritual offers a different form of self-care: Outside, putting one foot in front of the other, I connect with my surroundings, myself, family, and, on occasion, friends.

"The ability to take a walk from one point to the next point, that is half the battle won," the exuberant illustrator Maira Kalman scrawls in her marvelous book *My Favorite Things*, ingeniously capturing the experience. Alongside a painting of yellow flats with white bows, she adds: "Go out and take a walk. That is the glory of life."

As you establish your walking ritual, you'll figure out what makes it most wondrous for you. Do you like to pick your route beforehand or do you enjoy the spontaneity of turning left or right whenever the mood strikes? Are you fueled by listening to the soft hush of the morning or do you prefer to get lost in whatever's playing in your headphones? Do you want to walk at a fast or slow pace? And you'll start to notice the surprises that lie in store—nature's shifting form, the people you bump into, the ideas that pop into your head.

Getting Some Fresh Air

As to the nitty-gritty of when and where to walk, here are suggestions to help you get out the door:

- Walk right after you wake up. Use the bathroom, brush your teeth, throw on some clothes, and head out with your dog or yourself.

- Walk your child to school and take the long way back.

- Add extra walking time on your commute, either by getting off at an earlier bus or train stop or by parking farther from your destination.

- Meet a friend for a morning walk instead of a morning coffee.

- Take a midmorning walk break at work.

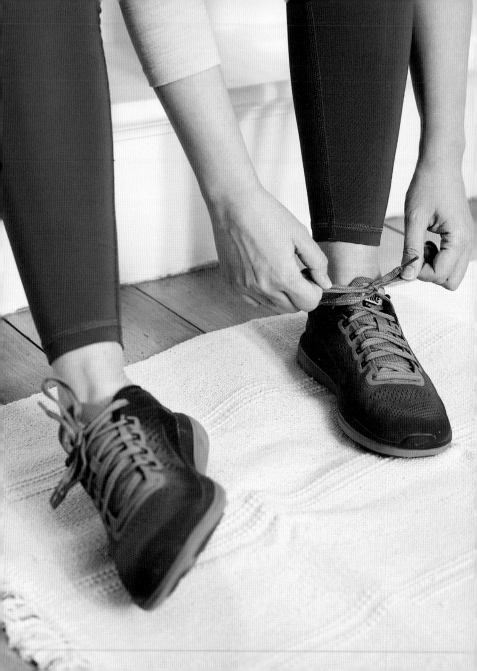

. . . or Going for a Run

When my younger daughter was two, I came down with chronic tonsillitis, which meant every six weeks I would have a high fever and feel like I was swallowing broken glass. One doctor told me I needed a tonsillectomy *stat*. Another informed me that she would have to be dragged by her arms and legs into the operating room, so painful is the recovery from the surgery as an adult. A third advised me to exercise more, because it was a good way to increase my immunity. With two small children and a job, I went for what seemed like the easiest option and laced up my sneakers.

And so, with the help of a "couch to 5K" app, I overcame my tonsillitis and slowly became a runner. And not just any runner! I turned into a smug, annoying runner—the kind who only wants to talk about how running cured her of getting sick. The first mile or so remained a slog, but then the endorphins kicked in, and even on the days I struggled to the last step, the end was glorious. It became a ritual. I run the exact same route every time, listening to the same songs over and over, through the heat and the cold.

Whether you want to train for a 5K or simply jog around the block a few times, making a ritual of it will only enhance the experience. As you put on your shoes, connect to your intention, to the idea that you are running toward discomfort—

possibly—but also flow. Heading out, recognize that you're part of a global community of runners. Welcome!

On the run itself, try repeating a mantra, something as simple as "I am a runner" or "Yes." And instead of obsessing about upping your speed or increasing your distance, take a moment to delight in your body's ability to move, propelled by your strength and determination. Afterward, pour yourself a big glass of water, sit still, and exult in the runner's high.

Tending to Your Plants

The taxi driver was lost—he'd warned us he hadn't heard of the place—so we told him to drop us by the dirt road. My husband and I were in the outskirts of Oaxaca, Mexico, searching for an orchid farm on our honeymoon. We weren't particularly interested in orchids or plants, but something about the description in the local tourist guidebook drew us to the place, so we trekked up the road. El Orquideario La Encantada—roughly translated as "the orchid garden under a spell"—has since become family lore.

When we finally found it, the owner, an architect who had given up his practice to cultivate a sanctuary for more than twelve hundred species of native orchids, handed us magnifying glasses and sent us exploring. We became so enchanted by the majesty of this secret garden and the vision of its creator, Octavio Gabriel Suárez, that we vowed to name any future son Octavio in his honor. In the end, while we only had daughters, we've paid tribute to his Eden by filling our home with plants inside and out. On summer mornings I relish stepping onto the terrace and tending to the plants in our little green patch.

You don't need to create a botanical garden to experience the incredible power of the plant world. Caring for just one fern can provide joy. Or you could experiment with growing

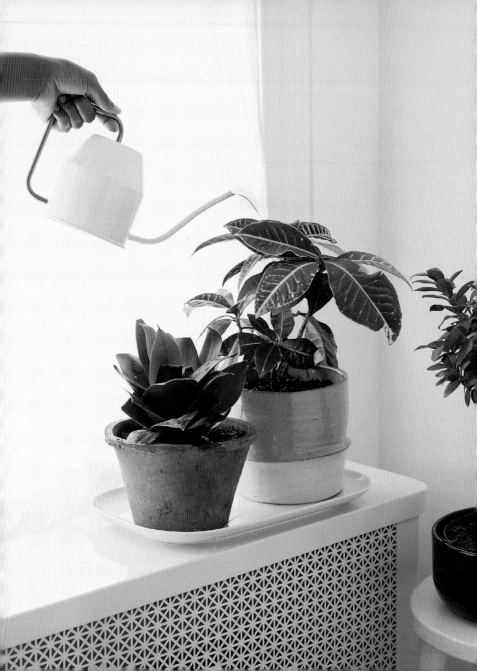

your own herbs—next thing you know, you'll be snipping the leaves from the small mint plant by the window for your nighttime tea or cutting chives for your lunch. Using one ritual to enhance another makes for an all-the-more-ritualistic lifestyle.

Your morning plant care ritual is rooted in creating a connection with living things, which means the specifics will necessarily shift depending on your plants' needs. Choose a route around your home or garden, and observe each plant, talk to them (research shows they will grow faster, especially if they hear a woman's voice), and give them love and encouragement. Some days you will water one or the other, some days you will prune leaves, some days you will rotate a pot's position toward the sun.

One last thing—the notion that some people are blessed with a green thumb and others are not leaves no space for learning and growing. No matter what color your thumb, gardening and plant care include moments of failure and disappointment as part of the life cycle. On the other side is the incredible wonder of watching something you potted and prune thrive.

Meditating

At the ages of seventy-nine and eighty-six, respectively, my mom and dad started meditating every morning. My mom told me that during one meditation, she felt a connection with her father who died from a heart attack when she was eight, allowing her to "finally mourn a little." About a month later, my dad called to console me about some disappointing news, explaining that he'd learned that "it was okay to feel sad." I was amazed by both my parents, but I was not surprised that meditation had opened them to new insights.

My own meditation practice has transformed the way I move through the world. I learned to notice my thoughts and actions instead of just getting lost in the narrative and, as a result, became less reactive and more compassionate toward myself and others. It started with a weekly meditation group after drop-off at my older daughter's elementary school. We parents would sit together for ten or fifteen minutes, sometimes guided, often not. That alone had such a positive impact on my well-being that I yearned for a deeper practice which, over the ensuing years, took the form of daily fifteen-minute meditations, loving-kindness meditations, meditation classes, and silent retreats to more deeply experience the joy and challenge of being mindful.

And yet, from time to time, for reasons I can't totally explain, I find myself taking a break from meditating. Funnily enough, I was in an off-period when my parents found the practice. This is to say, all of these things are true: Anyone can meditate, meditating is powerful, and still it's sometimes ridiculously hard to show up and do it. But, as my parents learned, creating a ritual around it makes meditating much easier. Here's one way to get there:

1 First, find the right time in *your* morning. There's a lot of advice out there suggesting that you roll straight out of bed and get meditating, but I've found that I'm in a much better mind-set after some caffeine. This is just another example of how important it is to tune in to what works for you, even if it differs from the standard doctrine.

2 Sit wherever you like: on the floor, the couch, a chair. My dad is not assuming Lotus Pose, and neither need you. Get comfortable.

3 Set a timer for however long you want. It can be one minute, it can be twenty-plus. (And it can change.)

4 Close your eyes and pay attention to your breath. I hated meditation when I first tried because the

teacher told us to focus on the sensation of our breath at the nose and I couldn't really feel it. Years later when I tried again, I found it much easier to pay attention to my chest rising and falling. If the breath isn't your jam, listen to the sounds in the room.

5   Accept that your mind will wander. This doesn't mean you're not doing it right! When you realize that you've gotten lost in thought, just go back to focusing on your breath or the room sounds. Expect this to happen again and again. This is meditating.

6   When the timer sounds, slowly open your eyes and look around. Pay attention to how your mind and body feel. (Congratulations! You're a meditator.)

Meditating on the Move

If you have trouble sitting down to meditate, you might try this alternative. I will warn you that it can feel pretty strange at first—it's definitely not your average walkabout, just with more mindfulness! When I first tried the formal practice on retreat, I felt self-conscious, but in subsequent experiences I have come to appreciate the focus it delivers.

To start, find a spot, either inside or out, where you won't be disturbed. Stand still and notice the physical aspects of doing so—the weight in your feet, the muscles holding you upright. Your hands can be in any comfortable position. Rather than focusing on your breath or the sounds around you, you're training your mind on the sensations in your body.

Then, take about a dozen slow steps. As you begin, pay attention to each step—lifting your foot, moving it forward, placing it down, shifting the weight. Notice any feelings of heaviness, lightness, or tingling in your body. Stay present for each step along the path. Just like in seated meditation, your mind will wander. Simply note any thoughts and return to the sensations in your body.

When you get to the end, pause and feel yourself standing in place before turning around and repeating the same deliberate process on the way back.

Reading a Poem

"The breeze at dawn has something to tell you. Don't go back to sleep," wrote the thirteenth-century poet Rumi. Eight hundred years later, Mary Oliver begins her poem "Why I Wake Early" with the line "Hello, sun in my face," and ends it with "Watch, now, how I start the day in happiness, in kindness." William Stafford woke daily at four a.m. to write his sixty-five volumes. Billy Collins asks, "Why do we bother with the rest of the day," in his aptly titled poem "Morning." The tie between the first hours of the day and poetry is clearly strong, and since poets are guides to the world, they must be on to something.

And so, let's turn to poems for language, rhythm, emotion, ideas, and observations as we start each and every day. Poetry is company for our hearts, a fast track into our interconnectedness with other beings and the natural world, a glimpse into the unknown, a shift of understanding and, above all, a gift for our spirit.

Luckily, adding a poetry ritual to your routine is quite easy. After meeting an old farmer whose grandfather had read poems out loud every morning to wake all the children in the house, the poet Naomi Shihab Nye started doing the same for her teenage son. She told Krista Tippett, host of the podcast *On Being*, how it transformed this otherwise mundane parenting task: "It was a pleasure, to me, to hear poems in the air first thing in the morning, by saying them to our beloved son." You can do the same for yourself (or another person in your house) by signing up for the Academy of American Poets' poem-a-day email, and a new poem, selected by a series of guest editors, will be delivered to your inbox around six a.m. This is a nice way to deepen your knowledge of different poets.

Or for a more tactile, off-screen experience (generally a plus with rituals), choose an anthology featuring many poems or a volume or two from one poet. If you don't know any, I think the aforementioned wordsmiths are all wonderful, as are Lucille Clifton, Rita Dove, Ocean Vuong, Joy Harjo, Donald Hall, Sharon Olds, Claribel Alegría. . . . This is my list, but you will make yours. Keep the volume near your bed and open it before you get dressed, or put it in your bag and read a poem on the train or sitting in the car, right before you go into the office. Let the words swirl around in your mouth and your mind and watch how they sustain you in unexpected ways throughout the day.

Greening Your Shower

Before forest bathing became a "thing" here in the United States, I stood under a canopy of trees in the Adirondack Mountains and actually showered. Looking above the hilltop cedarwood enclosure, I watched branches and leaves sway as birds sang and a cool breeze mixed with the heated mountain spring water pounding on my body. I wanted it to last forever, and since it couldn't, I spent the five-hour ride home fantasizing about traveling the world to document the most beautiful outdoor showers. Alas, the great majority of my showers since have been in my windowless bathroom, but a few eucalyptus branches perched atop the showerhead let me imagine I'm somewhere greener. Their scent clears my lungs and my mind, helping me step into the new day with a fresh perspective. This is how easy it is to make it happen:

1 Get a fresh eucalyptus bundle. You can often find them at farmers' markets, Trader Joe's, and flower shops. I change mine every four days or so.

2 Pound the leaves with a mallet to activate the scent.

3 Hang the bundle from your showerhead, using twine or a rubber band.

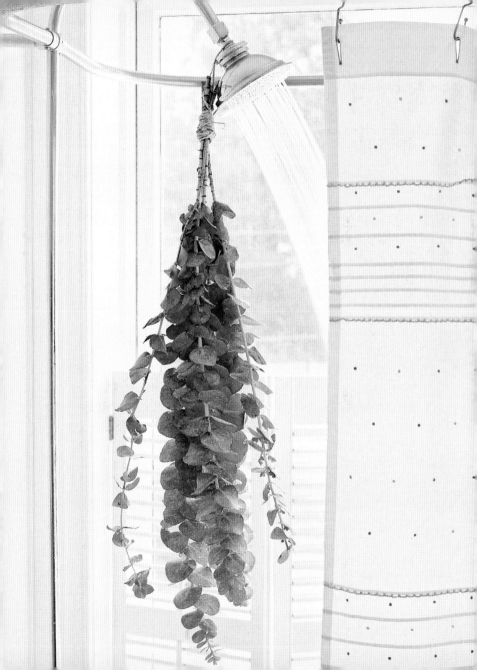

Braving the Cold

Fortune favors the bold. —Latin proverb

Better to not overthink this one. Just turn the shower knob to cold—slow and steady at first—and get your body under the freezing water. Head as well, please! Cold-shower evangelists will tell you that this brisk ritual can ease sadness, improve immunity, prevent migraines, repair muscles, and make skin glow. Whether or not that happens for you, I can say for certain that it will wake you up like nothing else.

Here's what to expect: You might scream, or yelp, but that's okay—let it out! Your body is in shock. Your breath will quicken. Your heart rate will get faster as blood rushes throughout your body. This will be hard, but you are reminded, right there under the freezing stream, that you can do hard things. Maybe you'll only stay for thirty seconds at first. Nevertheless, you'll have done it—you've challenged yourself, and the day's only just begun. This is reason enough.

Once you've worked your way up to evangelist status, decide whether you prefer to start warm and then go cold or brave the chill from the start—some people lather, shave, and shampoo under the arctic temps. Add a stretch to really rouse yourself, bending down to touch your toes and then reaching your arms to the sky, or incorporate the invigorating body scrub on the opposite page into your routine every few days.

Invigorating Citrus Body Scrub

Apply this energizing sugar scrub with a circular motion to exfoliate your skin and awaken your senses. Use it once or twice a week to avoid irritation. **MAKES ABOUT 1 CUP (285 G)**

1 cup (210 g) cane sugar
¼ to ⅓ cup (60 to 80 ml) coconut oil
Citrus essential oil (orange, lemon, or a mix)
Orange or lemon zest (optional)

Mix the sugar and coconut oil together (if the latter is solid, heat it for 10 seconds in the microwave to soften). Experiment with what consistency you prefer—I like it less oily, but you may prefer a little more. Put in a few drops of essential oil to begin, adding more for a stronger scent. Stir in the zest, if using. Massage a small scoop into your body, taking care to not scrub too hard, especially if you have sensitive skin.

Eating a Mindful Breakfast

A of lot us grow up reading the back of the cereal box during breakfast. In adulthood, our mealtime entertainment usually graduates to social media feeds, the news, or television. The downside is that we learn to pay little attention to what we are actually doing—eating. Likely that's why, some years ago, I realized I was scarfing down whatever was on my plate. This seemed an odd turn of events considering that when I wasn't eating, I gave significant headspace to food: thinking about what to eat, gathering the ingredients and preparing the meal or choosing the perfect restaurant for a night out. I felt I was missing out on a more nourishing and delicious culinary experience and decided to shift my habits, beginning at the breakfast table.

I turned to a Buddhist-inspired practice called mindful eating, which essentially teaches you to pay attention to each bite: noticing the flavors, sensations, and textures of a meal and any feelings that arise. Though this seems simple enough, I initially found it quite challenging and craved other input— but there were rewards for pushing through. I actually tasted what I ate! And I realized things about myself: for example, that I'm much happier and more sated if there's a crunchy element to my meal. A few years into this experiment, I can't claim to eat mindfully every morning, but I can say that I don't distract myself nearly as much.

If you've had a similar experience, follow these guidelines for your own mindful breakfast, which can take anywhere from ten to fifteen minutes:

1. Silence and put away all devices, and sit down at a table or counter where you can eat quietly and comfortably. Put your food on a nice plate or bowl.

2. Activate your senses: Look at what you're about to eat, noticing its colors and shape. Smell the food. Close your eyes and take a bite, paying attention to the flavors and texture, how it feels in your mouth, where you experience the flavor. Chew slowly.

3. Keep eating slowly, and notice your mind making judgments (*I'd rather be looking through my feed*), wandering (*What should I have for lunch?*), or experiencing emotions (*I shouldn't eat this food*). You're not doing anything wrong. Just as in meditation (see page 66), this mind drifting is natural. It's hard to teach your brain to focus on one thing! As soon as you realize it's happening, be kind to yourself and return your attention to eating.

A word of caution: Mindful eating is sometimes touted as a weight-loss trick, but that approach forces judgment and triggers emotions. The only goal here is to become more aware of, and present for, the experience of eating itself.

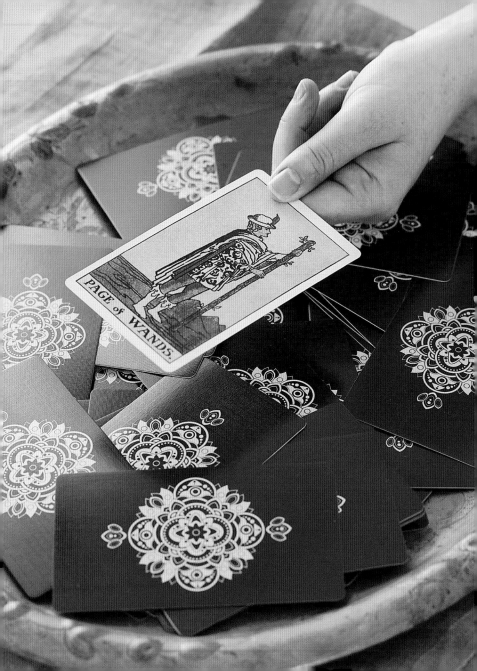

Pulling a Card

In my early thirties I became a devotee of a yoga studio on the eleventh floor of a former warehouse building. Sun streamed in through huge east-facing windows, lighting up the large white room like the slice of heaven it was to me. After years of trying yoga, I'd finally found a spot where my body and I connected. The teacher's instructions focused on alignment rather than racing from pose to pose, and this approach opened my poses and my heart. At the front of the room, there was a small brass bowl filled with the Original Angel Cards— little rectangular cards featuring a watercolor image of an angel (or two) and one inspirational word, such as *surrender*, *creativity*, or *kindness*. After I rolled up my mat, I made a ritual of slowly wandering up to the bowl—eagerly anticipating what message would come my way—and picking a card. I'd turn the word around in my mind, primed for any additional insights after an intense yoga practice.

For your own daily dose of guidance, start by finding a deck that really speaks to you. There are many choices, from traditional tarot to more open-ended oracle decks. With tarot, although the particular imagery might shift, a specific card's meaning is generally standard across decks. The best-known dates back more than a hundred years—Arthur E. Waite, a spiritual seeker and author, hired illustrator

Pamela Colman Smith, believing she was clairvoyant; their collaboration resulted in the iconic Rider-Waite-Smith cards. Oracle decks are far less prescribed. You can be guided by the moon, gods and goddesses, different spirits and energies, witches, art, animals, affirmations, poetry, angels . . . each has its own operating theory and significance. There are many beautiful options available online and at bookstores, gift shops, and metaphysical stores.

Some people, just before they pick a card, ask the deck a question they're seeking to answer. Others take a big breath and open their mind to whatever will come. Shuffle the cards until it feels like time to stop, then pick the one your hand gravitates toward. There are two ways to interpret your card: Tune in to your innate wisdom to find the message or guidance, or look to any accompanying guide for external input. Experiment to see what feels best.

Giving to Charity

Among all the rituals in this book, this one, which is focused on giving to others, may seem the most selfless. But I'd argue just the opposite—being of service is a salve for the soul. In that sense, it is the ultimate act of self-care.

There's something particularly valuable about starting each day with a charitable action. No matter how little or how much you can afford to give, it's a reminder that you are part of a bigger world, one in which you can be a force of good. To make it effortless, buy or make a small charity box and place it wherever you leave your wallet and keys. Before you head out each day, drop in something—a quarter, a dollar, more. Don't get hung up on the amount. If you never carry cash, you can use an app to collect the money. (For example, create a Tip Yourself jar on the Earnin app.) At the end of each month, gather your contributions and donate them to a cause. Or, for a little twist, pick a different friend each month, explain your ritual, and ask them to decide the recipient for that month's collection.

Set Up Your Day

I think a lot about transitions—the times when we move from one activity or phase of the day to another. They are often overlooked, despite their effect on everything from your productivity to your mood. They tend to be challenging and require a lot of energy. Once again, rituals to the rescue. They smooth the way beautifully, so that transitions feel less arduous and more graceful. The ones on the following pages are designed to do just that, helping you embrace the shift from morning to the day ahead.

Blending Up Some Sunshine

We needed to refill our fun bucket—my little family just wasn't getting along well. So for our big summer vacation, we let the kids decide the destination. Their vote was immediate and unanimous: Hawaii. My husband and I weren't so keen—it's nearly five thousand miles (eight thousand kilometers) from New York, and certainly not the cheapest trip in the world! But we'd made the offer and had been saving for this trip, so off to the Big Island we went. And thank goodness, because not only did we reconnect with one another while swimming, hiking, and exploring, but we also landed in a tiny second-floor acai shack above Snorkel Bob's rental office, enjoying some of the tastiest berry bowls of our lives.

They fuel us still: Whenever we're in the doldrums, we reminisce about the amazing acai we ate while perched on rickety wooden stools, looking out at the Pacific. Every minute of the fourteen-hour flight was worth it—we all want to go back. Until we return, my younger daughter has committed to a daily East Coast acai ritual, guaranteed to deliver a morning boost of tropical sunshine and good vibes.

Acai Bowl

Dark purple acai berries, which come from palm trees in the Brazilian Amazon, are bursting with antioxidants. They are processed into a pulp and sold in packets, which you can find at Trader Joe's, Target, natural food stores, and other retailers. Make sure you are buying ones with no added sugar. SERVES 1

1 packet frozen acai

½ cup (75 g) frozen strawberries

½ frozen banana

½ cup (115 g) Greek yogurt

½ cup (120 ml) milk or milk alternative
   (such as oat or coconut milk)

OPTIONAL ADD-INS, FOR SERVING:

Granola

Sliced fresh fruit, such as berries and/or bananas

Honey

Coconut flakes

Rinse the acai packet under hot water for a few seconds until you can break it up a bit. Transfer the acai to a blender along with the frozen strawberries and banana, yogurt, and milk. Blend until smooth. Pour the mixture into a bowl and top with any add-ins you like—the more the merrier.

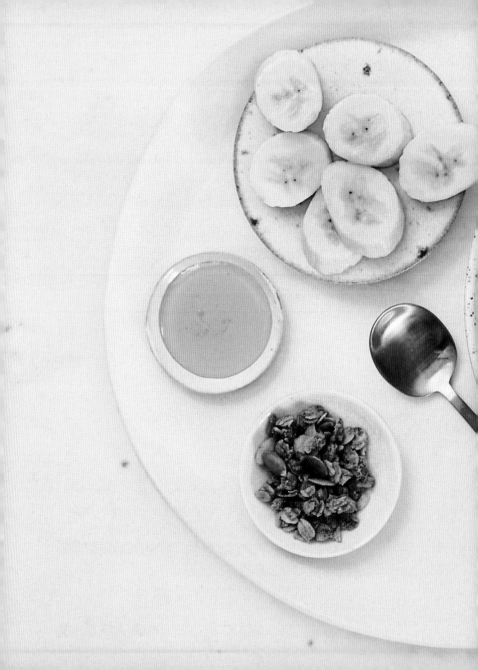

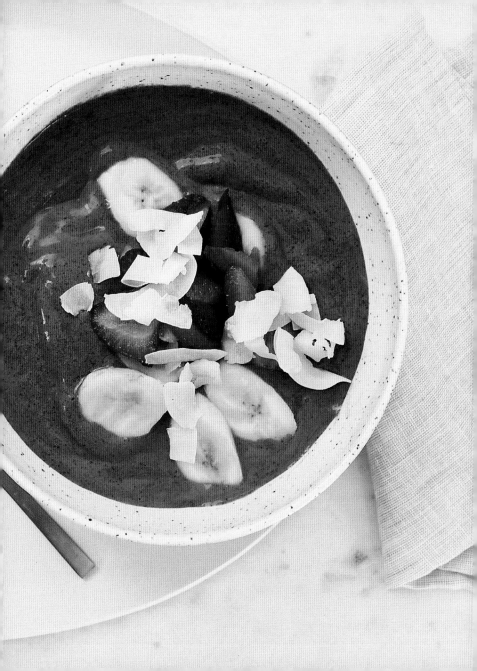

Writing a To-Do List

> *One morning Toad sat in bed.*
> *"I have many things to do," he said.*
> *"I will write them*
> *all down on a list*
> *so that I can remember them."*
> *Toad wrote on a piece of paper:*
> *A List of things to do today*
> *Then he wrote:*
> *Wake up*
> *"I have done that," said Toad,*
> *and he crossed out:*
> *Wake up*
> *Then Toad wrote other things on the paper.*

Thus starts one of my favorite stories about two dear
companions in *Frog and Toad Together* by Arnold Lobel. It's all
going well for Toad and his list; he gets through Eat Breakfast,
Get Dressed, and Go to Frog's House, but just after he crosses
off Take Walk with Frog, a strong wind blows the list out of
his hand. Frog urges Toad to run and catch it, but he can't:
"Running after my list is not one of the things that I wrote on
my list to do!" Frog runs over hills and swamps to try to catch

Toad's list, but alas, no luck. Toad, unable to remember any of the things on his list, decides he must sit and do nothing for the rest of the day.

Toad's right; it's overwhelming to keep track of the many things we must do. Even if our list flies away by midday—literally or metaphorically—there's value in having put it all down on paper. There are endless suggestions for how to do this most productively; let's explore how to do it ritually.

1 Find a paper you love: a personalized notepad, say, or heavy-stock rectangular cards. Whatever you plan to use, keep it somewhere within eyesight in the morning so you remember to write your list.

2 Use a special writing instrument: a prized fountain pen, gel pens, colored pencils.

3 Sit down, get quiet, and think about what you need and want to accomplish today.

4 To start, write: "Write my to-do list."

5 Consult yesterday's to-do list. If there is anything to carry over, write that. If there's an item that you keep carrying over, pause on it. Acknowledge that you're procrastinating. Maybe it's part of your process, or maybe you don't need to do it at all.

continued

6　When you finish writing your list, cross off "Write my to-do list."

7　Keep the list nearby, maybe in your pocket or phone case or taped to your computer.

8　If you realize you did something that you forgot to put on the list, it is absolutely legit to add it to your list and immediately cross it off. Credit where credit is due. This ritual is designed for maximum positive feedback loops and pats on the back.

By the way, it all works out for Toad in the end. As it gets late, Frog suggests that they go to sleep. Toad remembers that "Go to Sleep" was the last thing on his list, and, using a stick, writes, "Go to Sleep" on the ground before crossing it out and going to bed.

Listening to a Daily Anthem

My motto: When in doubt, Beyoncé.

I turn to Queen B to jump-start my morning—and pretty much everything else in my life. Another of my heroes, Serena Williams, reportedly walks onto the court listening to "Flashdance . . . What a Feeling." My beloved Michigan Wolverines have their fight song, "The Victors." Music is so energizing that years ago, marathon organizers tried to ban music devices to prevent, in part, plugged-in runners from having a competitive advantage.

Fortunately, you don't have to deal with any such regulations. You can tune out the rest of the world by tuning in to whatever beat will get you centered and prepped for the day. Find a time in the morning that works for you—before you head out, the last five minutes of the drive to the office, or the walk from the subway station all work—cue up your anthem, and let it fill your ears and lift your energy.

Caring for Your Skin

I belong to a family of beauty lovers. My granny whipped out her plastic rain bonnet at the first drop to protect her hairdo, my mom never left the house without "putting on her face," and my daughters are always trying new products. Me? I didn't get the gene—I'm lucky if I manage an SPF moisturizer, mascara, and lipstick. I used to sit in the bathroom and watch my mom do her makeup, applying each layer with care and precision. She had a lot on her plate—us kids, an aging mother, a sibling with intellectual disabilities, and a job—and this mirror time gave her the strength to face the world. As a kid, I mostly wanted her to hurry up, but as an adult I appreciate the value of her ritual.

Whether you have the beauty bug or not, there's a lot to be said for carving out a moment (or more) to care for yourself, even if it's just using a simple cleanser or running a jade roller over your cheeks. I always feel better when I've made the effort. Some days I take it a step further and dab on a face mask, enjoying the sensation of the creamy compound tightening on my skin, not to mention the tingle and glow after the fact. I've included a simple DIY recipe, opposite, so you can experience the same.

Bentonite Clay Mask

I use this mask whenever my face is starting to break out. Find the powdered clay, which is made from volcanic ash, in bulk online or in the beauty section of many natural food stores.

MAKES 1 MASK

1½ teaspoons (5 g) bentonite clay
1 teaspoon (5 ml) apple cider vinegar
1 teaspoon (5 ml) water

Mix the clay, vinegar, and water in a small bowl. Apply the mixture to your face, avoiding your eyes and mouth, and let it dry for 10 to 15 minutes. Wash off with a dampened cotton pad or soft washcloth, and pat your face dry.

Packing a Lunch

When I started packing a lunch for the office, it was for the virtuous reasons of saving money and eating healthier. Virtue only gets me so far, though. I keep packing my lunch because the ritual brings a mix of self-care and resourcefulness to my morning. After I make lunch for my kids, I get to work on mine—pivoting to my wants and needs is nourishing in itself. I also relish the constraints. As my designer friend Caroline says, "Creativity thrives in a sandbox." Lunch must consist of items on hand, stand up to travel, and, most essentially, taste good. This is not a sad desk lunch; it's a care package made with love.

And so I pull out the off-white ceramic bowl and its leakproof top, which I purchased specifically for this purpose. To keep things easy and efficient, the main ingredients for my lunch bowl are fairly straightforward: grains, potatoes, or greens combined with a protein. The meal shines because of the extras—something pickled, fresh herbs, nuts, cheese, or olives—and any premade dressing I have on hand, usually packed in its own small mason jar. The lids sealed and accomplishment noted, I place the goodies into a tote and finish getting ready for the day. All this prep has another, unintended, consequence: easing the transition from one mindset—home—to the next, so it's off to work I go.

A Lunch-Making Matrix

This ritual is easier to sustain if you have things on hand to mix and match. I make grains on the weekend, use leftovers from dinner, buy and make sauces, and use jarred pickled items. It's very flexible, which means I can assemble lunch quickly. You can pack the crispy items in a separate container and add them right before you eat for maximum crunchiness. I recommend getting yourself a light, leakproof container and metal utensils for easier transporting and more sustainable and luxurious lunching.

Base	Protein	Add-ins	Dressing	Crunch
Grains (white or brown rice, farro, quinoa)	Hard-boiled eggs	Cheese (my go-to is feta)	Dijon vinaigrette	Nuts or seeds
Potatoes (small and boiled, or roasted sweet potato wedges)	Tinned or cooked fish	Avocado	Olive oil and lemon juice	Raw vegetables (cucumbers, radishes, carrots)
	Shredded chicken	Vegetables like broccoli, spinach, cauliflower, beets (roasted, steamed, or sautéed)	Peanut sauce	Fried onions or shallots
Greens (something hearty like romaine lettuce, kale, even sautéed Brussels sprouts)	Legumes (black beans, chickpeas, lentils)		Soy-ginger sauce	Furikake seasoning
		Pickled items (sauerkraut, jalapeños, red onions)	Lemon-tahini dressing	Crumbled chips (plantain, tortilla)
		Fresh herbs	Pesto	

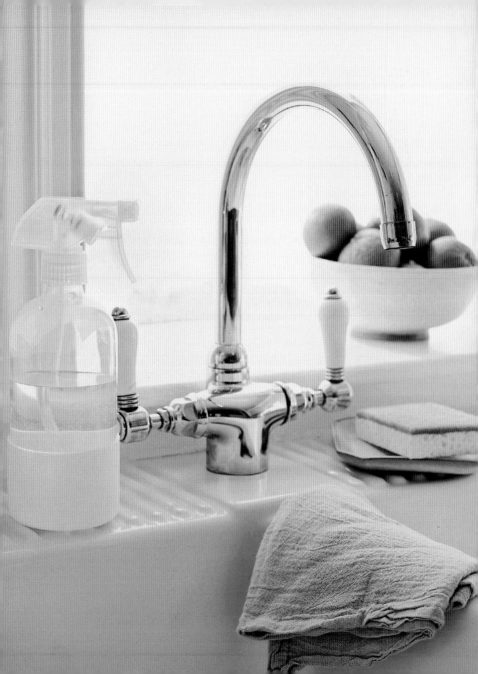

Tidying Up

Making your bed is the most heralded of all the morning rituals. The simple act of pulling up the covers, tucking in corners, and fluffing the pillows starts the day on the right foot, providing many people a quick hit of accomplishment and order. But, as my husband is fond of saying, I'm not one of those people. I make my bed when I remember, but I don't always remember. On the other hand, I hate starting my work day when my kitchen's a mess, so I always do the dishes—which, on days when I can wash them slowly, is both enjoyable at the time and results in a more pleasant scene when I return.

The question is: What do *you* need to do to get your home in order, in a way that makes you feel more harmonious in the moment and when you're going about your day? Whatever your answer—pulling up the shades, wiping the bathroom counter, putting away dirty clothes—it will be more satisfying if you do it joyfully, alert to the spiritual aspects of taking care of your home and possessions. Japanese Buddhist monks begin each day at their temple with *soji*, a twenty-minute cleaning ritual. "We don't do this because it's dirty or messy," writes Shoukei Matsumoto in *A Monk's Guide to a Clean House and Mind*. "We do it to eliminate the suffering in our hearts." The ritual opens up space in their minds, shows respect for their environment, and creates a connection with the world around them.

Improving Your Commute

I can trace my belief that small rituals improve daily life straight back to my father's forty-minute commute. Growing up, our home was filled with train chatter: which train Dad needed to make going in, which one he hoped to catch back, gripes from my brother and me when he missed the earlier one and we had to wait longer for dinner. But in the twenty years he commuted, I never heard a lot of complaints from him. On the contrary, even when it was crowded or delayed, his ride was a peaceful time—a few stolen moments between the demands of work and family. On the way in, he read the newspapers. Coming home, he worked until the train got two stops away, then he shut his eyes and napped for the final ten minutes. He walked through the door refreshed and happy—thanks, in part, to the seemingly small, inconsequential rituals that shaped his day and ours, turning what could have been a killjoy into the opposite.

What does this mean for your commute? Whether you're taking public transportation or driving, stalled trains, delayed buses, and morning traffic jams offer excellent, if unexpected, opportunities for mindfulness. Turn off any music or podcasts you are listening to, state your intention to stay present, and tune in to the noises and vibrations around you. Pay attention to your breath, notice any thoughts and feelings that arise, then go back to the breath. Obviously, if you're driving, you'll need to watch the road, but staying present will help with this; rather than losing yourself in a mental argument or daydream, you'll be keenly aware of what's happening around you.

I've also used my commute to do a loving-kindness meditation, which means silently wishing the best for myself, those in my life, those around me, and those around the world. And if you want to go in a different direction, you can make a ritual of reading or listening to an audiobook or doing crosswords. The point is to be intentional, not just pass the time mindlessly scrolling through your phone. Whichever route you choose, here are a few additional tips:

Leave early: Give yourself the gift of some extra wiggle room. Even the best ritual will be more challenging if you're stressed about time.

Have compassion: If someone cuts off your car or takes the last seat, try to recognize your shared humanity. It may calm you to remember that the people around you are in the same boat—just trying to get to work. It's not you against them.

Expect the unexpected: Annoying things will happen, with regularity. Remember that it's not personal. It's life. (The 4-7-8 breath ritual described on page 29 will be very helpful here!)

Arriving in Your Day

I can't say for sure how much of my worldview I owe to Fred Rogers, but I hope it's a lot. My brother and I were such devotees of *Mister Rogers' Neighborhood* that once, after watching Mr. Rogers visit a barber, my brother ran past my mom, grabbed scissors, and chopped off a big chunk of his own hair, all the way down to the scalp. Unfortunate haircuts aside, we were lucky to grow up watching Mr. Rogers. He modeled kindness and the importance of listening, and he celebrated the same small, everyday moments that I'm championing here in this book.

There's a lot of advice about how to start your day to ensure maximum productivity. And to be honest, part of me felt compelled to offer you the same get-up-and-go magic. But I kept thinking about Mr. Rogers's daily arrival on our television screen. He'd walk into his living room, hang up his blazer, zip up his cardigan, sit down to take off his fancy shoes, slip on his sneakers, and tie the laces. There was nothing high powered about this ritual, but he'd go on to make so much happen— he tackled topics like war, divorce, and racism. He made generations of children feel seen and worthy, and he took us to my most favorite place, the Neighborhood of Make Believe.

Wherever you're landing for the day after the big morning push, whether it's your home office, a playground with your child, an early morning class, or your desk at work, I hope you'll also grant yourself a slow, peaceful moment to honor the transition. As Mr. Rogers famously said, "How many times have you noticed that it's the little quiet moments in the midst of life that seem to give the rest extra-special meaning?" Say good morning to your colleague, hang up your coat, grab a glass of water, make a cup of coffee, unpack your bag, take out your to-do list, wipe your desk, eat a piece of fruit, stack your papers, read the news, review your goals, sit down, take a breath. . . . Do whatever it is that will settle your spirit so you can go on to have a beautiful—and impactful—day in your neighborhood.

Further Reading

The Artist's Way by Julia Cameron
The bible on writing morning pages
and the creative process.

Breath by James Nestor
An in-depth exploration of the
importance of proper breathing,
including specific exercises.

**Daily Rituals: How Artists Work
and Daily Rituals: Women at Work
by Mason Currey**
Detailed accounts of the rituals of those
who've accomplished great things:
Agatha Christie, Alexander Graham
Bell, Nikki Giovanni, and the like.

Every Body Yoga by Jessamyn Stanley
Practical information and inspiration
for both experienced and aspiring yogis
of all shapes and sizes.

**A Fearless Heart by Thupten
Jinpa, PhD**
A discourse on living with intention
and compassion from a former monk.

How to Meditate by Pema Chödrön
A clear exploration of the basics of
meditation for those who want to start
or deepen their practice.

**How to Wash the Dishes
by Peter Miller**
A small, pretty tome that elevates
this mundane duty into something
thoughtful and intentional.

**A Monk's Guide to a Clean House
and Mind by Shoukei Matsumoto**
This Japanese best-seller offers a
mindful approach to cleaning your
house and spirit.

A Thousand Mornings by Mary Oliver
Poems from the late Pulitzer Prize
winner, who had a morning ritual of
heading out at dawn with her pen and
notebook.

When by Daniel H. Pink
An argument for doing certain things
at specific times of the day, with advice
on maximizing your mornings.

**A Year of Mornings by Maria
Alexandra Vettese and Stephanie
Congdon Barnes**
Visual documentation of the morning
photography ritual of two women who
live 3,191 (5,135 km) miles apart.

Acknowledgments

What a privilege it was to write this book. I'm grateful for the opportunity to share these ideas with readers like yourself, and also for the following people, who helped bring it to life:

Bridget Monroe Itkin, for the collaboration of my dreams. Thank you for seeing the possibilities and trusting me with your vision, for being kind, empowering, and thoughtful, and for the perfect edits and Zoom backgrounds. Lia Ronnen, publisher extraordinaire, and the amazing Artisan team: Carson Lombardi, Suet Chong, Jane Treuhaft, Erica Heitman-Ford, Paula Brisco, Annie O'Donnell, Nancy Murray, Hanh Le, Allison McGeehon, Theresa Collier, Amy Michelson, and Patrick Thedinga.

Alexandra Grablewski for the lovely photographs; Maeve Sheridan and Cyd Raftus McDowell for the gorgeous styling. Models Iman Young, Kiah Stern, and Suet Chong. And Diana Mejia for the wonderful illustrations.

Gary Belsky, your friendship is foundational and transformative. To you and the best surprise, Neil Fine: I'm the luckiest that you let me worm my way into Elland Road Partners and tap into your magic. For your unconditional support, ideas, tweaks, endless verbal processing, and good snacks. Thank you for knowing me and having my back.

Kirkland Shephard and Shira Atkins, for your generosity and knowledge. For sharing rituals and insights, and enriching my life: Allisyn, Caroline K., Caroline R., Chelsea, Claudia, Cricket, Gundula, Holly, Jason, Jill, Jo, Keren, Lainie, Lauren, Lori, Margie, Rachel, Randy, Sam, Shira, and Stacey. Pam, the G's and I thank you and love you.

Mom and Dad. Brother. Martha and Agustín. Filippa, my fellow ritual girl, for our walks and talks. Lola, my kindred spirit, for reminding me of the power of stories. And Juan Pablo, por todo.

Finally, I wrote this book during the COVID-19 pandemic and want to acknowledge my dependence on, and gratitude for, the healthcare workers, the first responders, the scientists, the delivery people, the farm pickers, the grocery store workers, the teachers, the officials, and everyone else who put their lives at risk to show up. Thank you.

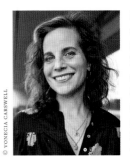

© VONECIA CARSWELL

Leslie Koren started her career as a local newspaper reporter, writing about everything from transportation issues to court proceedings before turning to more joyful matters: cooking, design, family, and happiness. In addition to *Morning Rituals*, she is the author of *Love Rituals* and *Restorative Rituals*. The former editor of *Crain's 5boros*, Leslie has written for various national and local publications. She lives in Brooklyn, New York, with her husband and two daughters.